Weight Loss Recipe Watchers 2025

Transform Your Kitchen & Your Body with Everyday Recipes That Make Weight Loss Simple, Sustainable and Delicious

By Author

Dr. Max K. Beck

Copyright © **Dr. Max K. Beck** 2025

All rights reserved. No part of this publication maybe reproduced, stored or transmitted in any form or by any means, electronic, mechanical, photocopying, recording, scanning, or otherwise without written permission from the author. It is illegal to copy this book, post it to a website, or distribute it by any other means without permission.

Dr. Max K. Beck

The moral right to be identified as the author of this work.

TABLE OF CONTENT

TABLE OF CONTENT	3
INTRODUCTION	6
BENEFITS OF THIS COOKBOOK	7
TIPS AND TRICKS FOR SUCCESS	7
ADVANTAGES OF THIS COOKBOOK OVER OTHERS	8
GRILLED LEMON HERB CHICKEN	9
ZUCCHINI NOODLES WITH PESTO	10
TURKEY AND VEGETABLE STIR-FRY	11
CAULIFLOWER CRUST PIZZA	12
SPINACH AND FETA STUFFED CHICKEN BREAST	13
6 SHRIMP AND BROCCOLI SKEWERS	14
QUINOA SALAD WITH ROASTED VEGETABLES	15
SWEET POTATO AND BLACK BEAN CHILI	16
GREEK YOGURT PARFAIT WITH BERRIES	17
BAKED SALMON WITH DILL SAUCE	18
EGG WHITE VEGETABLE OMELETTE	18
12 TURKEY AND QUINOA MEATBALLS	19
BUTTERNUT SQUASH SOUP	21
LEMON GARLIC SHRIMP SKEWERS	21
VEGGIE-LOADED TURKEY TACOS	22
SKINNY CHICKEN ALFREDO:	23
CUCUMBER AND TOMATO SALAD	24
BLACKENED TILAPIA WITH MANGO SALSA	25
CHICKPEA AND SPINACH CURRY	26
BAKED COD WITH LEMON DIJON GLAZE	27
CAPRESE STUFFED PORTOBELLO MUSHROOMS	29
TURKEY AND SWEET POTATO HASH	30
BROCCOLI AND CHEDDAR STUFFED CHICKEN	31
SHRIMP AND AVOCADO SALAD	32
LENTIL AND VEGETABLE SOUP	33
GRILLED VEGETABLE QUESADILLAS	34

- TERIYAKI CHICKEN LETTUCE WRAPS 35
- CAULIFLOWER FRIED RICE 36
- LEMON HERB QUINOA BOWL 37
- MEDITERRANEAN CHICKPEA SALAD 38
- BAKED BUFFALO CAULIFLOWER BITES 39
- LEMON GARLIC ROASTED BRUSSELS SPROUTS 40
- TUSCAN WHITE BEAN SOUP 41
- PESTO ZOODLES WITH CHERRY TOMATOES 42
- ASIAN GINGER GARLIC CHICKEN 43
- STUFFED BELL PEPPERS WITH GROUND TURKEY 44
- LEMON ROSEMARY ROASTED CHICKEN 45
- TURKEY AND VEGETABLE SKILLET 46
- CABBAGE AND APPLE SLAW 47
- BAKED TERIYAKI SALMON 48
- GREEK TURKEY BURGERS WITH TZATZIKI 49
- SOUTHWEST QUINOA BOWL 50
- BBQ CHICKEN LETTUCE WRAPS 51
- RATATOUILLE WITH QUINOA 51
- LEMON THYME GRILLED SHRIMP 52
- TURKEY AND BLACK BEAN ENCHILADAS 53
- CUCUMBER DILL GREEK YOGURT SALAD 54
- SWEET AND SOUR CHICKEN STIR-FRY 55
- CAULIFLOWER AND BROCCOLI GRATIN 56
- TOMATO BASIL ZUCCHINI NOODLES 58
- MOROCCAN CHICKPEA STEW 59
- BALSAMIC GLAZED CHICKEN BREAST 60
- PESTO TURKEY MEATLOAF 61
- SHRIMP AND ASPARAGUS STIR-FRY 62
- CHICKEN AND VEGETABLE KEBABS 63
- ROASTED RED PEPPER HUMMUS STUFFED CHICKEN 64
- QUINOA AND BLACK BEAN STUFFED PEPPERS 65
- TERIYAKI TOFU LETTUCE WRAPS 66

ITALIAN TURKEY AND VEGETABLE SOUP	67
LEMON GARLIC ROASTED SALMON	68
SPINACH AND MUSHROOM EGG MUFFINS	69
TURKEY AND SWEET POTATO SKILLET	70
GREEK QUINOA SALAD	71
BAKED EGGPLANT PARMESAN	72
CHICKEN AND BROCCOLI QUICHE	73
PESTO SHRIMP AND ZUCCHINI NOODLES	74
SPICY BLACK BEAN AND CORN SALSA	75
LEMON HERB GRILLED SWORDFISH	76
MEDITERRANEAN STUFFED BELL PEPPERS	77
THAI COCONUT CURRY CHICKEN	78
CAPRESE CHICKEN SKEWERS	79
CAULIFLOWER AND CHICKPEA CURRY	80
TURKEY AND SPINACH STUFFED MUSHROOMS	81
ASIAN SESAME SALMON BOWL	82
ZUCCHINI AND CORN FRITTERS	83
CONCLUSION	84

INTRODUCTION

Greetings from the Weight Loss Recipe Book for Watchers, your reliable guide to a more energetic, healthy version of yourself. This cookbook offers tasty, simple-to-make dishes that fit your objectives and lifestyle, whether you're just beginning your weight loss journey, returning after a hiatus, or need some new motivation to keep going.

Eating bland, uninteresting food, restricting one, or depriving one are not effective ways to lose weight. It's about striking a balance, savoring your food, and consistently choosing foods that fuel your body and promote your health. You'll genuinely look forward to eating the clever, tasty, low-point meals in this book, which range from filling lunches and energizing breakfasts to cozy dinners and guilt-free desserts.

All of the recipes have been carefully created with ease of use and delight in mind. You won't need to spend hours in the kitchen or use sophisticated ingredients. Instead, you'll find real-food recipes that you can easily incorporate into your daily routine, whether you're preparing meals for the coming week, cooking for one person, or feeding your family.

The tried-and-true ideas of points-based eating, which emphasize deliberate decision-making and don't restrict any food, served as the inspiration for this cookbook. The recipes are made to allow you to enjoy substantial amounts and strong flavors without going over your daily allotment. You'll find a wide range of meals that demonstrate that you can eat healthily and lose weight at the same time, from inventive new favorites to lightened-up classics.

These pages also contain useful advice, useful substitutions, and suggestions for maintaining motivation even when life becomes hectic or the scale isn't moving as fast as you'd want. Because true success is about feeling good about your body, taking care of yourself, and forming enduring habits, not simply about numbers.

This cookbook is for you, regardless of your weight loss objectives—whether it's 10 pounds or 100—or just feeling stronger, more energized, and more in charge of your health. Allow it to motivate, inspire, and remind you that eating well can be flexible, happy, and genuinely fulfilling.

BENEFITS OF THIS COOKBOOK

Supports Sustainable Weight Loss: All recipes are designed to align with a points-based system (like WW), making it easier to stay within your daily limits without counting calories obsessively.

Reduces Mealtime Stress: With quick, simple recipes that use everyday ingredients, this cookbook takes the guesswork out of healthy eating—perfect for busy schedules.

Boosts Energy & Improves Health: By focusing on whole, nutrient-dense ingredients, these recipes help you feel full longer, curb cravings, and nourish your body.

Helps You Stay on Track: Each dish is created to be satisfying and low in points so you can enjoy a variety of meals while still making progress toward your goals.

Encourages Family-Friendly Eating: No need to cook separate meals! These recipes are delicious and appealing for the whole family—so you're not going on this journey alone.

TIPS AND TRICKS FOR SUCCESS

Meal Prep = Momentum: Prepare ingredients or full meals in advance to avoid impulsive, high-point choices when you're tired or busy.

Don't Fear Flavor: Use herbs, spices, lemon juice, vinegar, garlic, and broth to pack in flavor without adding points.

Bulk Up with Zero-Point Foods: Add veggies, lean proteins, or beans to stretch meals, make them more filling, and keep you satisfied.

Portion with Purpose: Use measuring cups or a food scale (especially early on) to learn proper serving sizes—it makes a big difference!

Plan you're Treats: Leave a few points for a treat you love each day. It's easier to stay on track when you don't feel deprived.

Keep Staples Handy: Stock your pantry with healthy basics like canned beans, low-sodium broth, whole grains, frozen vegetables, and zero-sugar sauces.

ADVANTAGES OF THIS COOKBOOK OVER OTHERS

WW-Friendly Focus: Specifically designed with points-based eating in mind—no generic "diet food" here, just real meals that fit your goals.

No Complicated Ingredients: Every recipe uses accessible, budget-friendly ingredients you can find in any grocery store.

Versatile for All Lifestyles: Whether you're cooking for one, feeding a family, or prepping lunches for the week—there's something for every schedule.

Balanced & Satisfying: Recipes are designed to include protein, fiber, and healthy fats, helping you stay fuller longer and curb emotional eating.

Proven Weight Loss Support: Based on real-world strategies that align with how successful long-term weight loss really works: flexibility, enjoyment, and consistency.

GRILLED LEMON HERB CHICKEN

Servings: 4

Prep Time: 15 min

Cook Time: 15 min

Ingredients:

- 4 boneless, skinless chicken breasts
- 2 lemons (juiced)
- 3 tbsp olive oil
- 2 cloves garlic (chop-up)
- 1 tsp dried oregano
- 1 tsp dried thyme
- Salt and pepper as needed

Instructions:

1. Mix the lemon juice, olive oil, garlic, thyme, oregano, and salt and pepper in a bowl.
2. Pour the marinade over the chicken breasts and place them in a plastic bag that can be sealed. After sealing the bag, chill it for a minimum of 60 min.
3. Set the grill's temperature to medium-high.
4. Cook the chicken for 6 to 8 min on every side, or until it's done.
5. Enjoy while hot!

Nutrition Info (per serving):

Calories: 250, Protein: 30g, Carbohydrates: 3g, Fat: 12g

ZUCCHINI NOODLES WITH PESTO

Servings: 2

Prep Time: 10 min

Cook Time: 5 min

Ingredients:

- 2 medium zucchinis
- 1 cup of fresh basil leaves
- 1/4 cup of pine nuts
- 2 cloves garlic
- Half a cup of Parmesan cheese that has been finely grated
- 1/3 cup of olive oil
- Salt and pepper as needed

Instructions:

1. Zest the zucchini into spirals to make noodles.
2. Garlic, Parmesan, pine nuts, and basil should all be mixed in a food processor. Pulse until chop-up lightly.
3. Olive oil should be added gradually while the processor is running to fully blend the pesto.
4. For three to five min, toss zucchini noodles with pesto in a skillet over medium heat.
5. Toss as needed and season with salt and pepper.

Nutrition Info (per serving):

Calories: 300, Protein: 8g, Carbohydrates: 10g, Fat: 25g

TURKEY AND VEGETABLE STIR-FRY

Servings: 3

Prep Time: 20 min

Cook Time: 15 min

Ingredients:

- 1 lb lean ground turkey
- 2 cups of broccoli florets
- 1 bell pepper, split
- 1 cup of snap peas
- 2 carrots, julienned
- 3 tbsp low-sodium soy sauce
- 1 tbsp sesame oil
- 1 tbsp ginger, chop-up
- 2 cloves garlic, chop-up

Instructions:

1. Brown the ground turkey over medium-high heat in a sizable wok or skillet.
2. Stir-fry the garlic and ginger for one to two min.
3. Add the carrots, snap peas, bell pepper, and broccoli. Stir-fry for a further five to seven min.
4. Pour over the mixture with the soy sauce and sesame oil, tossing to thoroughly coat and cook.
5. Warm up the food.
6.

Nutrition Info (per serving):

Calories: 320, Protein: 25g, Carbohydrates: 15g, Fat: 18g

CAULIFLOWER CRUST PIZZA

Servings: 2

Prep Time: 20 min

Cook Time: 25 min

Ingredients:

- 1 medium cauliflower head, finely grated
- 1 egg
- 1 cup of part-skim mozzarella cheese, shredded
- 1 tsp dried oregano
- 1/2 tsp. garlic powder
- 1/4 cup of tomato sauce
- 1/2 cup of cherry tomatoes, split
- Tear-full 1/4 cup of basil

Instructions:

1. Turn the oven on to 425°F.
2. Finely grated cauliflower should be placed in a bowl that is safe to microwave for five min.
3. After letting the cauliflower cool, use a fresh kitchen towel to squeeze out any extra liquid.
4. Mix the cauliflower, egg, mozzarella, garlic powder, and oregano in a bowl.
5. On a baking sheet covered with paper, press the mixture into the shape of a pizza.
6. Bake crust till brown, 15 to 18 min.
7. Cover the crust with tomato sauce, then sprinkle basil and tomatoes over top.
8. Bake for a further ten to fifteen min.
9. Cut and savor!

Nutrition Info (per serving):

Calories: 280, Protein: 20g, Carbohydrates: 20g, Fat: 15g

SPINACH AND FETA STUFFED CHICKEN BREAST

Servings: 4

Prep Time: 15 min

Cook Time: 25 min

Ingredients:

- 4 boneless, skinless chicken breasts
- 2 cups of fresh spinach, chop up
- 1/2 cup of feta cheese, crumbled
- 2 cloves garlic, chop-up
- 1 tsp dried oregano
- Salt and pepper as needed

Instructions:

1. Set oven temperature to 375°F.
2. Add the chop-up spinach, feta, oregano, garlic, salt, and pepper to a bowl.
3. Cut every chicken breast in half horizontally to create a pocket.
4. Stuff the spinach and feta mixture inside every chicken breast.
5. After the chicken is cooked through, place the packed chicken breasts in a baking tray and bake for 25 min.
6. Warm up the food.

Nutrition Info (per serving):

Calories: 280, Protein: 35g, Carbohydrates: 3g, Fat: 12g

6 SHRIMP AND BROCCOLI SKEWERS

Servings: 4

Prep Time: 20 min

Cook Time: 10 min

Ingredients:

- Peeled and deveined big shrimp, around 1 pound
- 2 cups of broccoli florets
- 2 tbsp olive oil
- 1 tsp lemon zest
- 2 tbsp lemon juice
- 1 tsp garlic powder
- Salt and pepper as needed
- Wooden skewers, soaked in water

Instructions:

1. Set the grill's temperature to medium-high.
2. Shrimp, broccoli, olive oil, lemon zest, lemon juice, garlic powder, salt, and pepper should all be mixed in a bowl. Toss in the coat.
3. Put broccoli and shrimp on skewers.
4. Broccoli should be soft and shrimp opaque after 3–4 min on every side of the grill.
5. Warm up the food.

Nutrition Info (per serving):

Calories: 220, Protein: 25g, Carbohydrates: 6g, Fat: 10g

QUINOA SALAD WITH ROASTED VEGETABLES

Servings: 6

Prep Time: 15 min

Cook Time: 25 min

Ingredients:

- 1 cup of quinoa, rinsed
- 2 cup of cherry tomatoes, halved
- 1 zucchini, diced
- 1 red bell pepper, diced
- 1 red onion, split
- 2 tbsp olive oil
- 1 tsp dried thyme
- Salt and pepper as needed
- 1/4 cup of feta cheese, crumbled

Instructions:

1. Set oven temperature to 400°F.
2. Follow the directions on the package to cook the quinoa.
3. Mix cherry tomatoes, bell pepper, red onion, and zucchini in a bowl and toss to coat with olive oil, thyme, salt, and pepper.
4. Arrange the veggies onto a baking sheet and roast for twenty-five min, or until they become soft.
5. Roasted veggies and cooked quinoa should be mixed in a big bowl. Add feta on top if you'd like.
6. Warm or room-temperature servings are preferred.

Nutrition Info (per serving):

Calories: 280, Protein: 8g, Carbohydrates: 35g, Fat: 12g

SWEET POTATO AND BLACK BEAN CHILI

Servings: 8

Prep Time: 15 min

Cook Time: 30 min

Ingredients:

- 2 sweet potatoes, peeled and diced
- Then grab a can of black beans and rinse it well.
- 1 can (15 oz) diced tomatoes
- 1 onion, diced
- 3 cloves garlic, chop-up
- 1 tbsp chili powder
- 1 tsp cumin
- 1/2 tsp smoked paprika
- Salt and pepper as needed
- 4 cups of vegetable broth

Instructions:

1. Add the onion and garlic to a large pot and sauté until softened.
2. Add the diced tomatoes, black beans, sweet potatoes, cumin, smoked paprika, chili powder, and salt and pepper.
3. After adding the vegetable broth, boil the mixture. Cook until sweet potatoes are soft, 25 to 30 min.
4. Serve hot, adjusting the seasoning as necessary.

Nutrition Info (per serving):

Calories: 220, Protein: 8g, Carbohydrates: 45g, Fat: 2g

GREEK YOGURT PARFAIT WITH BERRIES

Servings: 2

Prep Time: 10 min

Cook Time: 0 min

Ingredients:

- 2 cups of Greek yogurt
- 1 cup of mixed berries
- 1/4 cup of granola
- 2 tbsp honey
- Mint leaves for garnish (non-compulsory)

Instructions:

1. Arrange Greek yogurt, mixed berries, and granola into two glasses or bowls.
2. Pour some honey on top.
3. If desired, garnish with mint leaves.
4. Serve right away.

Nutrition Info (per serving):

Calories: 250, Protein: 20g, Carbohydrates: 35g, Fat: 5g

BAKED SALMON WITH DILL SAUCE

Servings: 4

Prep Time: 10 min

Cook Time: 15 min

Ingredients:

- 4 salmon fillets
- 2 tbsp olive oil
- 2 tbsp lemon juice
- 1 tsp dried dill
- Salt and pepper as needed
- 1/2 cup of Greek yogurt
- 1 tbsp fresh dill, chop-up
- Lemon wedges for serving

Instructions:

1. Set oven temperature to 400°F.
2. Salmon fillets should be put on a baking pan. Pour in some lemon juice and olive oil. Dress with pepper, salt, and dried dill.
3. Bake the salmon for 12 to 15 min, or until it flakes easily with a fork.
4. Mix Greek yogurt and fresh dill in a small bowl.
5. Serve the salmon with lemon wedges and a dab of dill sauce.

Nutrition Info (per serving):

Calories: 300, Protein: 25g, Carbohydrates: 3g, Fat: 20g

EGG WHITE VEGETABLE OMELETTE

Servings: 2
Prep Time: 10 min
Cook Time: 10 min

Ingredients:

- 1 cup of egg whites
- 1/2 cup of bell peppers, diced
- 1/4 cup of red onion, diced
- 1/4 cup of tomatoes, diced
- 1/4 cup of spinach, chop up
- Salt and pepper as needed
- 1 tbsp olive oil
- Non-compulsory: 1/4 cup of feta cheese, crumbled

Instructions:

1. Whisk the egg whites, tomatoes, red onion, bell peppers, and spinach together in a bowl. Add pepper and salt for seasoning.
2. In a nonstick skillet, warm the olive oil over medium heat.
3. Once the edges are set, pour the egg mixture into the skillet and cook.
4. Using a spatula, gently lift the edges so that the raw egg can slide below.
5. Fold or flip the omelet in half once it's mostly set.
6. Cook for a further two to three min, or until well cooked.
7. Add some feta cheese on top before serving, if desired.

Nutrition Info (per serving):

Calories: 150, Protein: 20g, Carbohydrates: 6g, Fat: 5g

12 TURKEY AND QUINOA MEATBALLS

Servings: 4

Prep Time: 15 min

Cook Time: 20 min

Ingredients:

- 1 lb ground turkey
- 1 cup of cooked quinoa
- 1/4 cup of breadcrumbs
- 1 egg
- 2 cloves garlic, chop-up
- 1 tsp dried oregano
- Salt and pepper as needed
- 1 cup of tomato sauce

Instructions:

1. Set oven temperature to 375°F.
2. Ground turkey, cooked quinoa, breadcrumbs, egg, oregano, garlic, and salt and pepper should all be mixed in a bowl.
3. Place the meatballs you formed from the mixture onto a baking sheet.
4. Bake for 18 to 20 min, or until thoroughly done.
5. Cooked meatballs are added to a pan of heated tomato sauce.
6. Warm up the food.

Nutrition Info (per serving):

Calories: 280, Protein: 25g, Carbohydrates: 15g, Fat: 12g

BUTTERNUT SQUASH SOUP

Servings: 6

Prep Time: 15 min

Cook Time: 30 min

Ingredients:

- 1 butternut squash, peeled and diced
- 1 onion, chop-up
- 2 carrots, chop-up
- 2 apples, peeled and chop-up
- 1 tsp curry powder
- 1/2 tsp ground cinnamon
- 4 cups of vegetable broth
- Salt and pepper as needed
- 1/2 cup of Greek yogurt (for garnish)

Instructions:

1. Saute onion in a big pot until it becomes transparent.
2. Add the apples, carrots, butternut squash, cinnamon, curry powder, and salt & pepper. Simmer for five min.
3. After adding the veggie broth, bring it to a boil. Vegetables should simmer for 20 to 25 min to become soft.
4. Puree the soup in a blender until it's smooth.
5. Top with a dollop of Greek yogurt and serve hot.

Nutrition Info (per serving):

Calories: 150, Protein: 4g, Carbohydrates: 35g, Fat: 1g

LEMON GARLIC SHRIMP SKEWERS

Servings: 4

Prep Time: 15 min
Cook Time: 5 min

Ingredients:

- Peeled and deveined big shrimp, weighing 1 pound
- 2 tbsp olive oil
- 2 cloves garlic, chop-up
- 1 tsp lemon zest
- 2 tbsp lemon juice
- 1 tsp dried oregano
- Salt and pepper as needed
- Wooden skewers, soaked in water

Instructions:

1. Set the grill's temperature to medium-high.
2. Shrimp, olive oil, garlic, lemon zest, lemon juice, oregano, salt, and pepper should all be mixed in a bowl. Toss in the coat.
3. Assemble shrimp using skewers.
4. Grill until shrimp are opaque, 2 to 3 min per side.
5. Warm up the food.

Nutrition Info (per serving):

Calories: 180, Protein: 20g, Carbohydrates: 2g, Fat: 10g

VEGGIE-LOADED TURKEY TACOS

Servings: 4

Prep Time: 20 min
Cook Time: 15 min

Ingredients:

- 1 lb ground turkey
- 1 bell pepper, diced
- 1 zucchini, diced
- 1 cup of corn kernels
- One can of black beans who were just rinsed and drained
- 1 tbsp taco seasoning
- 8 whole wheat tortillas
- Toppings: shredded lettuce, diced tomatoes, salsa, Greek yogurt

Instructions:

1. Brown ground turkey over medium-high heat in a pan.
2. Add the taco spice, bell pepper, zucchini, corn, and black beans. Sauté the veggies until they are soft.
3. As directed on the package, warm the tortillas.
4. Place a spoonful of the turkey mixture on every tortilla.
5. Add Greek yogurt, salsa, chopped tomatoes, and shredded lettuce on top.
6. Present and savor!

Nutrition Info (per serving):

Calories: 300, Protein: 25g, Carbohydrates: 30g, Fat: 10g

SKINNY CHICKEN ALFREDO:

Servings: 4

Prep Time: 10 min

Cook Time: 20 min

Ingredients:

- 8 oz whole wheat fettuccine
- 1 lb boneless, skinless chicken breasts, thinly split
- 2 tbsp olive oil
- 3 cloves garlic, chop-up
- 1 cup of low-fat milk
- 1 cup of chicken broth
- 1 cup of finely grated Parmesan cheese
- Salt and pepper as needed
- 2 tbsp chop-up fresh parsley (for garnish)

Instructions:

1. Follow the directions on the package to cook the fettuccine.
2. Heat the olive oil in a pan over medium heat. Cook the chicken slices till they are browned.
3. Sauté the chop-up garlic for one to two min.
4. After adding the milk and chicken broth, boil the mixture.
5. Add Parmesan cheese and stir until smooth and melted.
6. Add pepper and salt for seasoning.
7. Add chop-up parsley as a garnish and toss the cooked fettuccine with the sauce.
8. Warm up the food.

Nutrition Info (per serving):

Calories: 450, Protein: 30g, Carbohydrates: 35g, Fat: 20g

CUCUMBER AND TOMATO SALAD

Servings: 4

Prep Time: 10 min
Cook Time: 0 min

Ingredients:

- 2 cucumbers, split
- 2 cup of cherry tomatoes, halved
- 1/2 red onion, thinly split
- 1/4 cup of feta cheese, crumbled
- 2 tbsp olive oil
- 1 tbsp red wine vinegar
- 1 tsp dried oregano
- Salt and pepper as needed
- Fresh basil leaves for garnish

Instructions:

1. Mix cucumbers, red onion, cherry tomatoes, and feta cheese in a big bowl.
2. Mix the olive oil, red wine vinegar, oregano, salt, and pepper in a small bowl.
3. Over the salad, drizzle with the dressing and toss to mix.
4. If desired, garnish with fresh basil leaves.
5. Present cold.

Nutrition Info (per serving):

Calories: 120, Protein: 3g, Carbohydrates: 10g, Fat: 8g

BLACKENED TILAPIA WITH MANGO SALSA

Servings: 4

Prep Time: 15 min

Cook Time: 10 min

Ingredients:

- 4 tilapia fillets
- 2 tsp paprika
- 1 tsp dried thyme
- 1 tsp onion powder
- 1 tsp garlic powder
- 1/2 tsp cayenne pepper
- Salt and pepper as needed
- 1 tbsp olive oil
- 1 mango, diced
- 1/2 red onion, lightly chop-up
- 1 jalapeño, seeded and diced
- 1/4 cup of fresh cilantro, chop up
- Juice of 1 lime

Instructions:

1. Mix the paprika, thyme, cayenne pepper, onion powder, garlic powder, and salt & pepper in a small bowl.
2. Coat the tilapia fillets on both sides with the spice mixture.
3. In a skillet set over medium-high heat, warm the olive oil. Cook tilapia for 3–4 min on every side, or until it's cooked through and browned.
4. To create the salsa, mix the mango, red onion, jalapeño, cilantro, and lime juice in a separate bowl.
5. Present the seared tilapia with a mango salsa on top.

Nutrition Info (per serving):

Calories: 220, Protein: 25g, Carbohydrates: 15g, Fat: 8g

CHICKPEA AND SPINACH CURRY

Servings: 4
Prep Time: 15 min
Cook Time: 25 min

Ingredients:

- 1 can (15 oz) chickpeas, drained and rinsed
- 1 onion, lightly chop-up
- 2 cloves garlic, chop-up
- 1 tbsp ginger, finely grated
- 1 tbsp curry powder
- 1 tsp ground cumin
- 1 tsp ground coriander
- 1/2 tsp turmeric
- 1 can (14 oz) diced tomatoes
- 1 can (14 oz) coconut milk
- 4 cups of fresh spinach
- Salt and pepper as needed
- Cooked brown rice for serving

Instructions:

1. Add the onion, garlic, and ginger to a large pot and sauté until softened.
2. Stir in turmeric, coriander, cumin, and curry powder. Simmer for one to two min.
3. Add the diced tomatoes, coconut milk, and chickpeas. Allow to simmer for fifteen min.
4. Cook the fresh spinach until it wilts.
5. Add pepper and salt for seasoning.
6. Place on top of warm brown rice.

Nutrition Info (per serving):

Calories: 320, Protein: 12g, Carbohydrates: 30g, Fat: 18g

BAKED COD WITH LEMON DIJON GLAZE

Servings: 4
Prep Time: 10 min
Cook Time: 20 min

Ingredients:

- 4 cod fillets
- 2 tbsp olive oil
- 2 tbsp Dijon mustard
- 1 tbsp honey
- 1 tbsp lemon juice
- 1 tsp dried thyme
- Salt and pepper as needed
- Lemon slices for garnish

Instructions:

1. Set oven temperature to 400°F.
2. Mix the olive oil, Dijon mustard, honey, lemon juice, thyme, salt, and pepper in a small bowl.
3. Cod fillets should be placed on a parchment paper-lined baking pan.
4. Apply the lemon-Dijon glaze to the fillets.
5. Bake for 18 to 20 min, or until a fork can easily pierce the fish.
6. Before serving, garnish with slices of lemon.

Nutrition Info (per serving):

Calories: 220, Protein: 25g, Carbohydrates: 5g, Fat: 10g

CAPRESE STUFFED PORTOBELLO MUSHROOMS

Servings: 2

Prep Time: 15 min

Cook Time: 20 min

Ingredients:

- 4 large Portobello mushrooms
- 1 cup of cherry tomatoes, split
- 1 cup of fresh mozzarella, diced
- 1/4 cup of fresh basil, chop up
- 2 tbsp balsamic glaze
- Salt and pepper as needed
- Olive oil for drizzling

Instructions:

1. Set oven temperature to 375°F.
2. After cleaning, cut off the stems from the Portobello mushrooms.
3. Cherry tomatoes, mozzarella, basil, balsamic glaze, salt, and pepper should all be mixed in a bowl.
4. Stuff the capers mixture into every mushroom.
5. After drizzling with olive oil, bake the mushrooms for 15 to 20 min, or until they are soft.
6. Warm up the food.

Nutrition Info (per serving):

Calories: 250, Protein: 15g, Carbohydrates: 10g, Fat: 18g

TURKEY AND SWEET POTATO HASH

Servings: 4

Prep Time: 15 min

Cook Time: 20 min

Ingredients:

- 1 lb ground turkey
- 2 sweet potatoes, peeled and diced
- 1 onion, diced
- 2 bell peppers, diced
- 2 cloves garlic, chop-up
- 1 tsp paprika
- 1 tsp ground cumin
- Salt and pepper as needed
- 2 tbsp olive oil
- Fresh parsley for garnish

Instructions:

1. In a pan set over medium-high heat, heat the olive oil.
2. Cook the ground turkey until it turns brown.
3. Add the bell peppers, onions, sweet potatoes, garlic, cumin, paprika, and salt & pepper.
4. Cook until the mixture is completely mixed and the sweet potatoes are soft.
5. If desired, garnish with fresh parsley.
6. Warm up the food.

Nutrition Info (per serving):

Calories: 320, Protein: 25g, Carbohydrates: 25g, Fat: 15g

BROCCOLI AND CHEDDAR STUFFED CHICKEN

Servings: 4

Prep Time: 15 min

Cook Time: 25 min

Ingredients:

- 4 boneless, skinless chicken breasts
- 1 cup of broccoli florets, steamed and chop-up
- 1 cup of cheddar cheese, shredded
- 2 tbsp cream cheese
- 1 tsp garlic powder
- 1 tsp onion powder
- Salt and pepper as needed
- Olive oil for drizzling

Instructions:

1. Set oven temperature to 400°F.
2. Slice every chicken breast in half lengthwise.
3. Mix broccoli, cheddar cheese, cream cheese, onion powder, garlic powder, salt, and pepper in a bowl.
4. Place a filling of the broccoli and cheddar mixture inside every chicken breast.
5. Once the chicken is cooked through, roast it for 20 to 25 min after drizzling it with olive oil.
6. Warm up the food.

Nutrition Info (per serving):

Calories: 300, Protein: 30g, Carbohydrates: 5g, Fat: 18g

SHRIMP AND AVOCADO SALAD

Servings: 2

Prep Time: 15 min

Cook Time: 0 min

Ingredients:

- Peeled and deveined big shrimp holding 1 pound
- 1 avocado, diced
- 1 cup of cherry tomatoes, halved
- 1 cucumber, diced
- 1/4 cup of red onion, lightly chop up
- 2 tbsp fresh cilantro, chop-up
- Juice of 2 limes
- 2 tbsp olive oil
- Salt and pepper as needed

Instructions:

1. Shrimp, avocado, cherry tomatoes, cucumber, red onion, and cilantro should all be mixed in a big bowl.
2. Mix the lime juice, olive oil, salt, and pepper in a small bowl.
3. After adding the dressing to the salad, gently toss to mix.
4. Present cold.

Nutrition Info (per serving):

Calories: 350, Protein: 25g, Carbohydrates: 15g, Fat: 22g

LENTIL AND VEGETABLE SOUP

Servings: 6

Prep Time: 15 min

Cook Time: 30 min

Ingredients:

- 1 cup of dried lentils, rinsed and drained
- 1 onion, chop-up
- 2 carrots, diced
- 2 celery stalks, diced
- 3 cloves garlic, chop-up
- 1 can (14 oz) diced tomatoes
- 6 cups of vegetable broth
- 1 tsp dried thyme
- 1 tsp ground cumin
- Salt and pepper as needed
- Fresh parsley for garnish

Instructions:

1. Lentils, chop-up tomatoes, celery, carrots, onion, garlic, cumin, thyme, and salt and pepper should all be mixed in a big pot.
2. Once the lentils are tender, simmer for 25 to 30 min on low heat after bringing to a boil.
3. As necessary, adjust the seasoning.
4. Before serving, garnish with fresh parsley.
5. Warm up the food.

Nutrition Info (per serving):

Calories: 250, Protein: 15g, Carbohydrates: 40g, Fat: 2g

GRILLED VEGETABLE QUESADILLAS

Servings: 4

Prep Time: 15 min

Cook Time: 15 min

Ingredients:

- 4 large whole wheat tortillas
- 1 zucchini, thinly split
- 1 red bell pepper, thinly split
- 1 yellow bell pepper, thinly split
- 1 red onion, thinly split
- 1 cup of mushrooms, split
- 1 cup of shredded mozzarella cheese
- 1 tbsp olive oil
- 1 tsp cumin
- Salt and pepper as needed
- Guacamole and salsa for serving

Instructions:

1. Set a grill pan or the grill to medium heat.
2. Mix the red, yellow, and green bell peppers, red onion, zucchini, and mushrooms in a bowl and toss with the olive oil, cumin, salt, and pepper.
3. Vegetables should be grilled until they are soft and have grill marks.
4. After the tortillas are arranged, evenly distribute the shredded mozzarella over everyone.
5. On one half of every tortilla, place the grilled vegetables, then fold the other half over.
6. Cook every quesadilla for two to three min on every side, or until the tortillas are crispy and the cheese is melted.
7. Serve hot with salsa and guacamole.

Nutrition Info (per serving):

Calories: 350, Protein: 15g, Carbohydrates: 45g, Fat: 12g

TERIYAKI CHICKEN LETTUCE WRAPS

Servings: 4

Prep Time: 20 min

Cook Time: 10 min

Ingredients:

- Diced chicken breasts that are 1 pound and free of bones and skin
- 1/4 cup of low-sodium soy sauce
- 2 tbsp honey
- 1 tbsp rice vinegar
- 1 tsp sesame oil
- 2 cloves garlic, chop-up
- 1 tsp ginger, finely grated
- 1 tbsp cornstarch
- 1 tbsp water
- 1 cup of water chestnuts, diced
- 1 cup of shiitake mushrooms, diced
- 1/4 cup of green onions, chop up
- Iceberg lettuce leaves for wrapping

Instructions:

1. Mix the sesame oil, honey, rice vinegar, ginger, garlic, and soy sauce in a bowl.
2. Cook the diced chicken in a skillet until it's browned and well done.
3. After adding the sauce, toss the chicken to coat.
4. Dissolve cornstarch in water in a small bowl. To thicken the sauce, add to the chicken mixture.
5. Add the green onions, shiitake mushrooms, and water chestnuts and stir.
6. Fill lettuce leaves with the chicken mixture using a spoon.
7. Serve right away.

Nutrition Info (per serving):

Calories: 280, Protein: 25g, Carbohydrates: 30g, Fat: 8g

CAULIFLOWER FRIED RICE

Servings: 4

Prep Time: 15 min

Cook Time: 15 min

Ingredients:

- 1 head cauliflower, finely grated or riced
- 2 tbsp sesame oil
- 1 cup of carrots, diced
- 1 cup of peas
- 2 eggs, beaten
- 3 green onions, chop-up
- 3 tbsp low-sodium soy sauce
- 1 tsp ginger, finely grated
- 1 tsp garlic, chop-up
- Salt and pepper as needed

Instructions:

1. Sesame oil should be heated over medium heat in a big skillet.
2. Add the peas and carrots, and sauté the veggies until they are soft.
3. Transfer the veggies to one side of the skillet and fill the space with the whisked eggs.
4. Add the scrambled eggs to the veggie mixture.
5. Stir in the garlic, ginger, soy sauce, green onions, and cauliflower rice. Blend thoroughly.
6. Cook the cauliflower for a further five to seven min, or until it is tender.
7. As needed, add salt and pepper for seasoning.
8. Warm up the food.

Nutrition Info (per serving):

Calories: 150, Protein: 8g, Carbohydrates: 20g, Fat: 6g

LEMON HERB QUINOA BOWL

Servings: 4

Prep Time: 10 min

Cook Time: 15 min

Ingredients:

- 1 cup ofquinoa, rinsed
- 2 cups of vegetable broth
- 1 lemon, juiced and zester
- 2 tbsp olive oil
- 1 tsp dried thyme
- 1 tsp dried rosemary
- 1 tsp dried parsley
- Salt and pepper as needed
- 1 cup of cherry tomatoes, halved
- 1 cucumber, diced
- 1/4 cup of feta cheese, crumbled

Instructions:

1. Mix the veggie broth and quinoa in a saucepan. Once the quinoa is done, bring it to a boil, then lower the heat and simmer for 15 min.
2. Mix lemon juice, zest, olive oil, thyme, rosemary, parsley, salt, and pepper in a bowl.
3. Using a fork, fluff the cooked quinoa before adding the herb and lemon dressing. To mix, toss.
4. Add the cucumber, feta cheese, and cherry tomatoes and fold gently.
5. Heat or serve at room temperature.

Nutrition Info (per serving):

Calories: 300, Protein: 8g, Carbohydrates: 40g, Fat: 12g

MEDITERRANEAN CHICKPEA SALAD

Servings: 4

Prep Time: 15 min

Cook Time: 0 min

Ingredients:

- 2 cans (15 oz every) chickpeas, drained and rinsed
- 1 cucumber, diced
- 1 cup of cherry tomatoes, halved
- 1/2 red onion, lightly chop-up
- 1/2 cup of Kalamata olives, split
- 1/2 cup of feta cheese, crumbled
- 1/4 cup of fresh parsley, chop up
- 2 tbsp extra virgin olive oil
- 1 tbsp red wine vinegar
- 1 tsp dried oregano
- Salt and pepper as needed

Instructions:

1. Chickpeas, cucumber, cherry tomatoes, red onion, olives, feta cheese, and parsley should all be mixed in a big bowl.
2. Mix the olive oil, red wine vinegar, oregano, salt, and pepper in a small bowl.
3. After adding the dressing to the salad, toss to mix.
4. Present cold.

Nutrition Info (per serving):

Calories: 320, Protein: 15g, Carbohydrates: 40g, Fat: 14g

BAKED BUFFALO CAULIFLOWER BITES

Servings: 4

Prep Time: 15 min

Cook Time: 25 min

Ingredients:

- 1 head cauliflower, cut into florets
- 1/2 cup of flour (can use almond flour for a gluten-free option)
- 1/2 cup of milk
- 1 tsp garlic powder
- 1 tsp onion powder
- 1/2 cup of buffalo sauce
- 2 tbsp melted butter
- Ranch

Instructions:

1. Set a baking sheet covered with parchment paper and preheat the oven to 450°F.
2. To make a batter, mix the flour, milk, onion powder, and garlic powder in a bowl.
3. Lay every cauliflower floret on the baking sheet that has been prepared after dipping it into the batter and allowing any excess drop-off.
4. Bake the cauliflower for 20 min, turning it over halfway through.
5. Mix melted butter and buffalo sauce in a different bowl.
6. Coat the cooked cauliflower thoroughly by tossing it in the buffalo sauce mixture.
7. Bake for five more min.
8. Serve hot with blue cheese or ranch dressing.

Nutrition Info (per serving):

Calories: 180, Protein: 5g, Carbohydrates: 20g, Fat: 10g

LEMON GARLIC ROASTED BRUSSELS SPROUTS

Servings: 4

Prep Time: 10 min

Cook Time: 20 min

Ingredients:

- 1 pound of Brussels sprouts, sliced finely
- 2 tbsp olive oil
- 3 cloves garlic, chop-up
- Zest of 1 lemon
- 1 tbsp lemon juice
- Salt and pepper as needed
- Parmesan cheese for garnish (non-compulsory)

Instructions:

1. Set a baking sheet covered with parchment paper and preheat the oven to 400°F.
2. Brussels sprouts should be mixed with olive oil, salt, pepper, lemon zest, and juice in a bowl.
3. Arrange the Brussels sprouts on the ready baking sheet.
4. Roast the Brussels sprouts for 20 min, or until they are crisp-tender and golden brown.
5. If desired, sprinkle some Parmesan cheese on top.
6. Warm up the food.

Nutrition Info (per serving):

Calories: 120, Protein: 5g, Carbohydrates: 15g, Fat: 6g

TUSCAN WHITE BEAN SOUP

Servings: 6

Prep Time: 15 min

Cook Time: 25 min

Ingredients:

- 2 tbsp olive oil
- 1 onion, chop-up
- 2 carrots, diced
- 3 cloves garlic, chop-up
- 2 cans (15 oz every) cannellini beans, drained and rinsed
- 4 cups of vegetable broth
- 1 tsp dried rosemary
- 1 tsp dried thyme
- 1 bay leaf
- Salt and pepper as needed
- 4 cups of fresh spinach
- 1/4 cup of fresh parsley, chop up

Instructions:

1. In a big pot, warm the olive oil over medium heat.
2. Add the carrots and onion, and chop-up. Sauté the food until it becomes tender.
3. Cook the chop-up garlic for one to two more min after adding it.
4. Add the bay leaf, rosemary, thyme, cannellini beans, vegetable broth, salt, and pepper.
5. After bringing the soup to a simmer, cook it for 15 to 20 min.
6. Add the parsley and fresh spinach. Cook until spinach starts to wilt.
7. Before serving, take the bay leaf off.
8. Warm up the food.

Nutrition Info (per serving):

Calories: 180, Protein: 8g, Carbohydrates: 30g, Fat: 4g

PESTO ZOODLES WITH CHERRY TOMATOES

Servings: 2

Prep Time: 10 min

Cook Time: 0 min

Ingredients:

- 4 medium zucchini, spiraled into zoodles
- 1 cup of cherry tomatoes, halved
- 1/2 cup of basil pesto
- 1/4 cup of pine nuts, toasted
- Finely grated Parmesan cheese for garnish
- Salt and pepper as needed

Instructions:

1. Toss zoodles with cherry tomatoes and basil pesto in a big bowl, being sure to coat them well.
2. As needed, add salt and pepper for seasoning.
3. Sprinkle finely grated Parmesan cheese and roasted pine nuts on top.
4. Serve right away.

Nutrition Info (per serving):

Calories: 300, Protein: 8g, Carbohydrates: 15g, Fat: 25g

ASIAN GINGER GARLIC CHICKEN

Servings: 4

Prep Time: 15 min

Cook Time: 20 min

Ingredients:

- 1 lb boneless, skinless chicken breasts, thinly split
- 2 tbsp soy sauce
- 1 tbsp hoisin sauce
- 1 tbsp rice vinegar
- 1 tbsp sesame oil
- 1 tbsp fresh ginger, finely grated
- 2 cloves garlic, chop-up
- 1 tbsp cornstarch
- 2 tbsp water
- 2 tbsp green onions, chop up
- Sesame seeds

Instructions:

1. Mix the rice vinegar, ginger, garlic, sesame oil, hoisin sauce, and soy sauce in a bowl.
2. Give the chicken slices at least ten min to marinate in the sauce.
3. Cook the marinated chicken in a skillet over medium-high heat until it's browned and well done.
4. Dissolve cornstarch in water in a small bowl. To make the sauce thicker, add to the skillet.
5. Add sesame seeds and green onions as garnish.
6. Serve hot with noodles or rice.

Nutrition Info (per serving):

Calories: 250, Protein: 25g, Carbohydrates: 8g, Fat: 12g

STUFFED BELL PEPPERS WITH GROUND TURKEY

Servings: 4

Prep Time: 20 min

Cook Time: 30 min

Ingredients:

- 4 Bell peppers, seeded and halved
- 1 lb lean ground turkey
- 1 cup of cooked quinoa
- 1 can of black beans that have been rinsed and drained
- 1 cup of corn kernels
- 1 cup of salsa
- 1 tsp cumin
- 1 tsp chili powder
- Salt and pepper as needed
- 1 cup of shredded cheddar cheese
- Fresh cilantro for garnish

Instructions:

- Set oven temperature to 375°F.
- Cook the ground turkey in a pan until browned.
- Cooked turkey, quinoa, black beans, corn, salsa, cumin, chili powder, salt, and pepper should all be mixed in a big bowl.
- The mixture should be spooned into the bell pepper halves.
- Put some shredded cheddar cheese on top of every stuffed pepper.
- Bake for 25 to 30 min, or until the cheese melts and the peppers become soft.
- Before serving, garnish with fresh cilantro.
- Warm up the food.

Nutrition Info (per serving):

Calories: 350, Protein: 25g, Carbohydrates: 30g, Fat: 15g

LEMON ROSEMARY ROASTED CHICKEN

Servings: 4

Prep Time: 10 min

Cook Time: 1 hr

Ingredients:

- 1 whole chicken
- 2 lemons, split
- 3 cloves garlic, chop-up
- 2 tbsp fresh rosemary, chop-up
- 2 tbsp olive oil
- Salt and pepper as needed

Instructions:

1. Set oven temperature to 375°F.
2. After rinsing, blot the chicken dry with paper towels.
3. Mix chop-up rosemary, olive oil, salt, and pepper in a small bowl along with chop-up garlic.
4. Apply the mixture of garlic and rosemary to the outside as well as the inside of the chicken.
5. Put slices of lemon inside the chicken's cavity.
6. Use kitchen thread to secure the chicken legs together.
7. Bake the chicken for approximately one hour, or until the internal temperature reaches 165°F, in the preheated oven.
8. Before slicing, give the chicken ten min to rest.
9. Warm up the food.

Nutrition Info (per serving):

Calories: 400, Protein: 30g, Carbohydrates: 2g, Fat: 30g

TURKEY AND VEGETABLE SKILLET

Servings: 4

Prep Time: 15 min

Cook Time: 20 min

Ingredients:

- 1 lb ground turkey
- 1 onion, chop-up
- 2 bell peppers, diced
- 2 zucchini, diced
- 2 cloves garlic, chop-up
- 1 tsp cumin
- 1 tsp chili powder
- 1 tsp paprika
- Salt and pepper as needed
- 1 can of black beans that have been rinsed and drained
- 1 cup of corn kernels
- 1 cup of salsa
- 1 cup of shredded cheddar cheese
- Fresh cilantro for garnish

Instructions:

1. Cook the ground turkey till browned in a large skillet.
2. Add the chop-up garlic, bell peppers, zucchini, and chop-up onion. Add the veggies and sauté until they soft.
3. Add salt, pepper, paprika, chili powder, and cumin for seasoning.
4. Add the salsa, corn, and black beans and stir. Cook until well heated.
5. Place shredded cheddar cheese on top of the griddle and let it melt.
6. Add fresh cilantro as a garnish.
7. Warm up the food.

Nutrition Info (per serving):

Calories: 300, Protein: 25g, Carbohydrates: 20g, Fat: 15g

CABBAGE AND APPLE SLAW

Servings: 4

Prep Time: 15 min

Cook Time: 0 min

Ingredients:

- 1/2 head of green cabbage, shredded
- 2 apples, julienned
- 1/2 cup of Greek yogurt
- 2 tbsp mayonnaise
- 1 tbsp Dijon mustard
- 1 tbsp honey
- 1 tbsp apple cider vinegar
- Salt and pepper as needed
- 1/4 cup of chop-up walnuts for garnish

Instructions:

1. Mix the julienned apples and the shredded cabbage in a big bowl.
2. Greek yogurt, mayonnaise, Dijon mustard, honey, apple cider vinegar, salt, and pepper should all be mixed in a small bowl.
3. Over the cabbage and apple combination, drizzle the dressing. For an even coat, toss.
4. Add chop-up walnuts as a garnish.
5. Present cold.

Nutrition Info (per serving):

Calories: 180, Protein: 3g, Carbohydrates: 25g, Fat: 8g

BAKED TERIYAKI SALMON

Servings: 4

Prep Time: 15 min

Cook Time: 15 min

Ingredients:

- 4 salmon fillets
- 1/4 cup of soy sauce
- 2 tbsp honey
- 1 tbsp rice vinegar
- 1 tbsp sesame oil
- 2 cloves garlic, chop-up
- 1 tsp ginger, finely grated
- Sesame seeds and chop-up green onions for garnish

Instructions:

1. Set a baking sheet covered with parchment paper and preheat the oven to 400°F.
2. To make the teriyaki sauce, mix the soy sauce, honey, rice vinegar, sesame oil, ginger, and garlic in a bowl.
3. Put the salmon fillets onto the baking sheet that has been prepared.
4. Saving some of the teriyaki sauce for later, brush it over the salmon.
5. Bake the salmon for 12 to 15 min, or until it is thoroughly done.
6. Before serving, drizzle with the remaining teriyaki sauce.
7. Add chop-up green onions and sesame seeds as garnish.
8. Warm up the food.

Nutrition Info (per serving):

Calories: 300, Protein: 25g, Carbohydrates: 15g, Fat: 15g

GREEK TURKEY BURGERS WITH TZATZIKI

Servings: 4

Prep Time: 20 min

Cook Time: 15 min

Ingredients:

- 1 lb ground turkey
- 1/2 cup of feta cheese, crumbled
- 1/4 cup of red onion, lightly chop up
- 1/4 cup of fresh parsley, chop up
- 1 tsp dried oregano
- Salt and pepper as needed
- 4 whole wheat burger buns
- Tzatziki sauce for serving
- Split cucumbers, tomatoes, and red onions for topping

Instructions:

1. Ground turkey, feta cheese, red onion, parsley, oregano, salt, and pepper should all be mixed in a bowl.
2. Create four burger patties out of the mixture.
3. The burgers should be cooked through after grilling or cooking them in a skillet over medium heat for about 6-7 min on every side.
4. Give the whole wheat buns a toast.
5. Top the turkey burgers with chop-up cucumbers, tomatoes, red onions, and tzatziki sauce and serve them on the buns.
6. Warm up the food.

Nutrition Info (per serving):

Calories: 350, Protein: 25g, Carbohydrates: 25g, Fat: 18g

SOUTHWEST QUINOA BOWL

Servings: 4

Prep Time: 15 min

Cook Time: 20 min

Ingredients:

- 1 cup ofquinoa, rinsed
- 2 cups of vegetable broth
- 1 can of black beans that have been rinsed and drained
- 1 cup of corn kernels
- 1 cup of cherry tomatoes, halved
- 1 avocado, diced
- 1/4 cup of red onion, lightly chop up
- 1/4 cup of fresh cilantro, chop up
- 1 lime, juiced
- 1 tsp ground cumin
- 1 tsp chili powder
- Salt and pepper as needed
- Greek yogurt

Instructions:

1. Mix the veggie broth and quinoa in a saucepan. Once the quinoa is cooked, bring it to a boil, then lower the heat and simmer for 15 to 20 min.
2. Cooked quinoa, black beans, corn, avocado, red onion, cilantro, lime juice, cumin, chili powder, salt, and pepper should all be mixed in a big bowl.
3. Mix the ingredients until thoroughly blended.
4. Spoon the quinoa mixture into bowls and garnish with a dollop of sour cream or Greek yogurt.
5. Warm up and serve.

Nutrition Info (per serving):

Calories: 300, Protein: 10g, Carbohydrates: 45g, Fat: 10g

BBQ CHICKEN LETTUCE WRAPS

Servings: 4

Prep Time: 15 min

Cook Time: 20 min

Ingredients:

- • Diced chicken breasts within 1 lb. with no evidence of bones & skin
- 1/2 cup of barbecue sauce
- 1 tbsp olive oil
- 1 red bell pepper, diced
- 1/2 red onion, lightly chop-up
- 1 cup of pineapple chunks
- 1/4 cup of fresh cilantro, chop up
- Iceberg lettuce leaves for wrapping

Instructions:

1. In a pan set over medium-high heat, heat the olive oil.
2. Cook the chop-up chicken until it turns brown.
3. Drizzle the chicken with barbecue sauce and toss to coat.
4. Add the diced pineapple chunks, red onion, and red bell pepper. Adjust oil & sauté veggies until soft. Add the chop-up cilantro and stir.
5. Divide the BBQ chicken mixture among the leaves of the iceberg lettuce.
6. Serve right away.

Nutrition Info (per serving):

Calories: 250, Protein: 20g, Carbohydrates: 25g, Fat: 8g

RATATOUILLE WITH QUINOA

Servings: 4
Prep Time: 20 min
Cook Time: 40 min

Ingredients:

- 1 eggplant, diced
- 2 zucchini, split
- 1 yellow bell pepper, diced
- 1 red onion, diced
- 2 cloves garlic, chop-up
- 1 can (15 oz) diced tomatoes
- 2 tbsp tomato paste
- 1 tsp dried thyme
- 1 tsp dried rosemary
- Salt and pepper as needed
- 1 cup of quinoa, rinsed
- 2 cups of vegetable broth
- Fresh basil for garnish

Instructions:

1. Chop-up eggplant, split zucchini, chop-up red onion, diced yellow bell pepper, chop-up garlic, diced tomatoes, tomato paste, thyme, rosemary, salt, and pepper should all be mixed in a big pot.
2. Stirring occasionally, simmer the mixture over medium heat for thirty to forty min.
3. Quinoa and vegetable broth should be mixed in a different saucepan. Once the quinoa is cooked, bring it to a boil, then lower the heat and simmer for 15 to 20 min.
4. Over cooked quinoa, serve ratatouille.
5. Throw some fresh basil on top.
6. Warm up and serve.

Nutrition Info (per serving):

Calories: 320, Protein: 10g, Carbohydrates: 60g, Fat: 5g

LEMON THYME GRILLED SHRIMP

Servings: 4

Prep Time: 15 min
Cook Time: 5 min

Ingredients:

- •Peeled and deveined big shrimp, weighing 1 lb.
- 2 tbsp olive oil
- 2 tbsp fresh lemon juice
- 1 tbsp fresh thyme leaves, chop-up
- 2 cloves garlic, chop-up
- Salt and pepper as needed
- Lemon wedges for garnish

Instructions:

1. Mix the olive oil, lemon juice, thyme, garlic, salt, and pepper in a bowl.
2. Toss to coat the shrimp after adding them to the marinade. Give it at least ten min to marinate.
3. Set the grill's temperature to medium-high.
4. Secure the shrimp with skewers.
5. Shrimp should be cooked through and opaque after grilling for two to three min on every side.
6. Zesty lemon wedges for garnish.
7. Warm up the food.

Nutrition Info (per serving):

Calories: 180, Protein: 20g, Carbohydrates: 2g, Fat: 10g

TURKEY AND BLACK BEAN ENCHILADAS

Servings: 4

Prep Time: 20 min
Cook Time: 25 min

Ingredients:

- 1 lb ground turkey
- 1 onion, chop-up
- 2 cloves garlic, chop-up
- 1 can of black beans that have been rinsed and drained
- 1 cup of corn kernels
- 1 tsp cumin
- 1 tsp chili powder
- Salt and pepper as needed
- 8 whole wheat tortillas
- 2 cups of enchilada sauce
- 1 cup of shredded cheddar cheese
- Fresh cilantro for garnish

Instructions:

1. Set oven temperature to 375°F.
2. Cook the ground turkey in a pan until browned. Add chopped garlic and diced onion. Once the onion is tender, sauté it.
3. Add the corn, black beans, chili powder, cumin, salt, and pepper and stir.
4. After reheating the tortillas, stuff everyone with the bean and turkey mixture.
5. The tortillas should be rolled up and put seam-side down in a baking dish.
6. Over the rolled tortillas, drizzle enchilada sauce and top with shredded cheddar cheese.
7. Bake the cheese for 20 to 25 min, or until it is bubbling and melted.
8. Before serving, garnish with fresh cilantro.
9. Warm up the food.

Nutrition Info (per serving):

Calories: 400, Protein: 25g, Carbohydrates: 35g, Fat: 18g

CUCUMBER DILL GREEK YOGURT SALAD

Servings: 4
Prep Time: 10 min
Cook Time: 0 min

Ingredients:

- 2 cucumbers, split
- 1 cup of cherry tomatoes, halved
- 1/2 red onion, thinly split
- 1/2 cup of Greek yogurt
- 1 tbsp olive oil
- 1 tbsp fresh dill, chop-up
- 1 tbsp lemon juice
- Salt and pepper as needed

Instructions:

1. Split red onion, cherry tomatoes, and cucumber slices should all be mixed in a big bowl.
2. Greek yogurt, olive oil, dill, lemon juice, salt, and pepper should all be mixed in a small bowl.
3. After adding the yogurt dressing, toss to coat the cucumber mixture.
4. Present cold.

Nutrition Info (per serving):

Calories: 100, Protein: 3g, Carbohydrates: 10g, Fat: 6g

SWEET AND SOUR CHICKEN STIR-FRY

Servings: 4
Prep Time: 15 min
Cook Time: 15 min

Ingredients:

- Cut up chicken breasts one lb wholly lacking in pieces & skin
- 1 cup of pineapple chunks
- 1 red bell pepper, split
- 1 green bell pepper, split
- 1 onion, split
- 1/2 cup of sweet and sour sauce
- 2 tbsp soy sauce
- 1 tbsp cornstarch
- 1 tbsp vegetable oil
- Cooked brown rice for serving
- Sesame seeds and split green onions for garnish

Instructions:

1. Mix soy sauce, cornstarch, and sweet and sour sauce in a bowl.
2. In a wok or sizable skillet, heat the vegetable oil over medium-high heat.
3. Stir-fry the chicken pieces until they are cooked through and golden.
4. To the wok, add pineapple chunks, onion, red and green bell peppers, and peppers. Stir-fry the veggies until they become crisp-tender.
5. Cover the chicken and veggies with the sauce. To coat, stir.
6. Simmer the sauce for a further two to three min, or until it thickens.
7. Overcooked brown rice, serve the sweet and sour chicken stir-fry.
8. Add split green onions and sesame seeds as garnish.
9. Warm up the food.

Nutrition Info (per serving):

Calories: 350, Protein: 25g, Carbohydrates: 30g, Fat: 12g

CAULIFLOWER AND BROCCOLI GRATIN

Servings: 4
Prep Time: 20 min
Cook Time: 25 min

Ingredients:
- 1 little head of cauliflower, cut in half into florets
- One little broccoli put, cut in half into florets
- 2 tbsp butter
- 2 tbsp all-purpose flour
- 2 cups of milk
- 1 cup of shredded cheddar cheese
- Finely grated Parmesan cheese, 1/4 cup
- 1 tsp Dijon mustard
- Salt and pepper as needed
- 1/4 cup of breadcrumbs
- Fresh parsley for garnish

Instructions:
1. Warm up the oven to 375°F and coat a baking dish with oil.
2. Broccoli and cauliflower should be steamed until just barely soft. Toss into the ready baking dish.
3. Melt butter in a pot over a medium heat. Add flour and stir to make a paste.
4. Add milk a little at a time, whisking until the mixture thickens.
5. Add salt, pepper, Dijon mustard, cheddar, and Parmesan cheese. Once the sauce is smooth and the cheeses have melted stir.
6. Cover the broccoli and cauliflower with the cheese sauce.
7. Mix the breadcrumbs and a little amount of melted butter in a small bowl, then sprinkle it on top.
8. Bake the gratin for 20 to 25 min, or until it's bubbling and brown.
9. Before serving, garnish with fresh parsley.
10. Warm up the food.

Nutrition Info (per serving):
Calories: 300, Protein: 15g, Carbohydrates: 25g, Fat: 16g

TOMATO BASIL ZUCCHINI NOODLES

Servings: 4

Prep Time: 15 min

Cook Time: 10 min

Ingredients:

- 4 medium zucchini, spiral zed into noodles
- 2 tbsp olive oil
- 3 cloves garlic, chop-up
- 1 pint cherry tomatoes, halved
- 1/4 cup of fresh basil, chop up
- Salt and pepper as needed
- Finely grated Parmesan cheese for garnish

Instructions:

1. In a big skillet put over medium heat, add the olive oil.
2. When aromatic, add the chop-up garlic and sauté it.
3. Cook the zucchini noodles for 3–4 min, or until they are just starting to soften.
4. Add the cherry tomatoes and simmer for a further two to three min.
5. Add pepper and salt for seasoning.
6. Add finely grated Parmesan cheese and chop up fresh basil as garnish.
7. Warm up the food.

Nutrition Info (per serving):

Calories: 80, Protein: 3g, Carbohydrates: 10g, Fat: 4g

MOROCCAN CHICKPEA STEW

Servings: 4
Prep Time: 20 min
Cook Time: 30 min

Ingredients:

- 2 tbsp olive oil
- 1 onion, chop-up
- 2 carrots, diced
- 2 cloves garlic, chop-up
- 1 tsp ground cumin
- 1 tsp ground coriander
- 1 tsp ground cinnamon
- 1 can (15 oz) chickpeas, drained and rinsed
- 1 can (15 oz) diced tomatoes
- 3 cups of vegetable broth
- 1 cup of butternut squash, diced
- 1/4 cup of dried apricots, chopped up
- Salt and pepper as needed
- Fresh cilantro for garnish

Instructions:

1. In a big pot, warm the olive oil over medium heat.
2. Add the diced carrots and onion. Sauté the food until it becomes tender.
3. Add the ground cinnamon, coriander, cumin, and chop-up garlic and stir.
4. Add the dried apricots, butternut squash, diced tomatoes, and vegetable broth to the chickpeas.
5. Add pepper and salt for seasoning. Heat through to a simmer.
6. When the vegetables are soft, around 25 to 30 min should pass, covered.
7. Before serving, garnish with fresh cilantro.
8. Warm up the food.

Nutrition Info (per serving):

Calories: 250, Protein: 8g, Carbohydrates: 40g, Fat: 8g

BALSAMIC GLAZED CHICKEN BREAST

Servings: 4

Prep Time: 10 min

Cook Time: 20 min

Ingredients:

- 4 boneless, skinless chicken breasts
- Salt and pepper as needed
- 1/4 cup of balsamic vinegar
- 2 tbsp honey
- 1 tbsp Dijon mustard
- 1 tbsp olive oil
- 2 cloves garlic, chop-up
- Fresh parsley for garnish

Instructions:

1. Set oven temperature to 400°F.
2. Add salt and pepper to chicken breasts for seasoning.
3. Mix the olive oil, honey, Dijon mustard, balsamic vinegar, and chopped garlic in a small bowl.
4. Transfer the chicken breasts to a baking dish and cover them with the balsamic glaze.
5. Bake the chicken for 20 min, or until it is thoroughly done.
6. Before serving, garnish with fresh parsley.
7. Warm up the food.

Nutrition Info (per serving):

Calories: 250, Protein: 30g, Carbohydrates: 10g, Fat: 10g

PESTO TURKEY MEATLOAF

Servings: 4

Prep Time: 15 min

Cook Time: 45 min

Ingredients:

- 1 lb ground turkey
- 1/2 cup of breadcrumbs
- 1/4 cup of pesto sauce
- Finely grated Parmesan cheese, 1/4 cup
- 1 egg
- 1/2 cup of milk
- Salt and pepper as needed
- Tomato sauce for topping

Instructions:

1. Grease a loaf pan and preheat the oven to 375 degrees.
2. Ground turkey, breadcrumbs, Parmesan cheese, pesto sauce, egg, milk, salt, and pepper should all be mixed in a big bowl.
3. Form into a loaf and place in the prepared pan after thoroughly mixing.
4. Cover the top of the meatloaf with tomato sauce.
5. Bake until the internal temperature reaches 165°F, about 45 min.
6. Before slicing, let it a few min to rest.
7. Warm up the food.

Nutrition Info (per serving):

Calories: 300, Protein: 25g, Carbohydrates: 15g, Fat: 15g

SHRIMP AND ASPARAGUS STIR-FRY

Servings: 4

Prep Time: 15 min

Cook Time: 10 min

Ingredients:

- 1 lb large shrimp, peeled and deveined
- One bunch of asparagus, rinsed and cut into 2-inch stems
- 2 tbsp soy sauce
- 1 tbsp oyster sauce
- 1 tbsp hoisin sauce
- 1 tbsp sesame oil
- 2 tbsp vegetable oil
- 2 cloves garlic, chop-up
- 1 tsp fresh ginger, finely grated
- Sesame seeds for garnish
- Cooked brown rice for serving

Instructions:

1. Mix the hoisin sauce, sesame oil, oyster sauce, and soy sauce in a bowl.
2. In a big skillet or wok, heat the vegetable oil over high heat.
3. Add the finely grated ginger and chop up garlic. For around 30 seconds, stir-fry.
4. Cook the shrimp until they become opaque and pink.
5. When the asparagus is crisp-tender, add it and stir-fry it for another two to three min.
6. Drizzle the asparagus and shrimp with the sauce. To coat, stir.
7. Simmer for a further one to two min, or until the sauce is thicker.
8. Add sesame seeds on top.
9. Overcooked brown rice, serve the stir-fried shrimp and asparagus.
10. Warm up the food.

Nutrition Info (per serving):

Calories: 250, Protein: 20g, Carbohydrates: 15g, Fat: 12g

CHICKEN AND VEGETABLE KEBABS

Servings: 4

Prep Time: 20 min

Cook Time: 15 min

Ingredients:

- 1 lb boneless, skinless chicken breasts, cut into chunks
- 1/2 a red bell pepper, cut
- 1 yellow bell pepper, cut into chunks
- 1 zucchini, split
- 1 red onion, cut into chunks
- 2 tbsp olive oil
- 2 tbsp balsamic vinegar
- 1 tsp dried oregano
- Salt and pepper as needed

Instructions:

1. Mix the olive oil, balsamic vinegar, salt, pepper, and dried oregano in a bowl.
2. Add bell peppers, zucchini, red onion, and chunks of chicken on skewers.
3. Apply the marinade that has been made to the kebabs.
4. Set the grill's temperature to medium-high.
5. Turn the kebabs once or twice while grilling them for ten to fifteen min, or until the chicken is cooked through and the veggies are soft.
6. Warm up the food.

Nutrition Info (per serving):

Calories: 250, Protein: 25g, Carbohydrates: 10g, Fat: 12g

ROASTED RED PEPPER HUMMUS STUFFED CHICKEN

Servings: 4

Prep Time: 15 min

Cook Time: 25 min

Ingredients:

- 4 boneless, skinless chicken breasts
- Salt and pepper as needed
- 1/2 cup of roasted red pepper hummus
- 1/4 cup of feta cheese, crumbled
- 1 tbsp olive oil
- Fresh parsley for garnish

Instructions:

1. Set oven temperature to 375°F.
2. Add salt and pepper to chicken breasts for seasoning.
3. Cut a horizontal incision to create a pocket in every chicken breast.
4. Mix feta cheese and roasted red pepper hummus.
5. Place a filling of feta and hummus inside every chicken breast.
6. In an oven-safe skillet, warm the olive oil over medium-high heat.
7. For two to three min on every side, sear the chicken breasts.
8. Place the skillet in the oven that has been preheated, and bake for 20 to 25 min, or until the chicken is thoroughly done.
9. Before serving, garnish with fresh parsley.
10. Warm up the food.

Nutrition Info (per serving):

Calories: 300, Protein: 30g, Carbohydrates: 4g, Fat: 18g

QUINOA AND BLACK BEAN STUFFED PEPPERS

Servings: 4

Prep Time: 15 min

Cook Time: 25 min

Ingredients:

- 4 Bell peppers, seeds and halved
- 1 cup of quinoa, cooked
- 1 can of black beans that have been rinsed and drained
- 1 cup of corn kernels
- 1 cup of salsa
- 1 tsp cumin
- 1/2 tsp chili powder
- Salt and pepper as needed
- 1 cup of shredded cheddar cheese
- Fresh cilantro for garnish

Instructions:

1. Set oven temperature to 375°F.
2. The cooked quinoa, black beans, corn, salsa, cumin, chili powder, salt, and pepper should all be mixed in a bowl.
3. Spoon the black bean and quinoa mixture into every side of a bell pepper.
4. Stuffed peppers should be put in a baking dish.
5. Place shredded cheddar cheese on top of every pepper.
6. The cheese should be melted and bubbling after 25 min in the oven.
7. Before serving, garnish with fresh cilantro.
8. Warm up the food.

Nutrition Info (per serving):

Calories: 350, Protein: 15g, Carbohydrates: 50g, Fat: 10g

TERIYAKI TOFU LETTUCE WRAPS

Servings: 4

Prep Time: 20 min

Cook Time: 10 min

Ingredients:

- 1 block firm tofu, drained and crumbled
- 1/4 cup of low-sodium soy sauce
- 2 tbsp teriyaki sauce
- 1 tbsp sesame oil
- 1 tbsp rice vinegar
- 1 tbsp honey
- 1 tbsp ginger, finely grated
- 1 clove garlic, chop-up
- 1 cup of shredded carrots
- 1/2 cup of chop-up green onions
- Butter lettuce leaves for wrapping
- Sesame seeds for garnish

Instructions:

1. Mix crumbled tofu, rice vinegar, teriyaki sauce, sesame oil, finely grated ginger, chopped-up garlic, and honey in a bowl.
2. For five to seven min, cook the tofu mixture in a pan over medium heat.
3. Add chop-up green onions and shredded carrots. Simmer for two more min.
4. Spoon the tofu mixture into the leaves of the butter lettuce.
5. Add sesame seeds as a garnish.
6. Serve right away.

Nutrition Info (per serving):

Calories: 180, Protein: 10g, Carbohydrates: 20g, Fat: 8g

ITALIAN TURKEY AND VEGETABLE SOUP

Servings: 4

Prep Time: 15 min

Cook Time: 30 min

Ingredients:

- 1 lb ground turkey
- 1 onion, chop-up
- 2 carrots, diced
- 2 celery stalks, diced
- 2 cloves garlic, chop-up
- 1 can (15 oz) diced tomatoes
- 4 cup of low-sodium chicken broth
- 1 cup of green beans, chop up
- 1 cup of zucchini, diced
- 1 tsp dried oregano
- 1 tsp dried basil
- Salt and pepper as needed
- Fresh parsley for garnish

Instructions:

1. Brown the ground turkey in a large pot over medium heat.
2. Add the chop-up garlic, diced celery, diced carrots, and split onion. Sauté the veggies till they get tender.
3. Add the diced tomatoes, chop-up green beans, diced zucchini, chicken broth, dried basil, dried oregano, and salt and pepper as needed.
4. The soup should be brought to a boil, then simmered for 20 to 25 min on low heat.
5. Before serving, garnish with fresh parsley.
6. Warm up the food.

Nutrition Info (per serving):

Calories: 280, Protein: 25g, Carbohydrates: 20g, Fat: 12g

LEMON GARLIC ROASTED SALMON

Servings: 4

Prep Time: 10 min

Cook Time: 15 min

Ingredients:

- 4 salmon fillets
- 2 tbsp olive oil
- 2 tbsp fresh lemon juice
- 2 cloves garlic, chop-up
- 1 tsp dried oregano
- Salt and pepper as needed
- Lemon slices for garnish

Instructions:

1. Set oven temperature to 400°F.
2. Mix olive oil, lemon juice, chopped garlic, dried oregano, salt, and pepper in a small bowl.
3. The salmon fillets should be put on a baking pan.
4. Apply the lemon-garlic mixture to the fish.
5. Bake the salmon for 12 to 15 min, or until it is thoroughly done.
6. Before serving, garnish with slices of lemon.
7. Warm up the food.

Nutrition Info (per serving):

Calories: 300, Protein: 25g, Carbohydrates: 1g, Fat: 20g

SPINACH AND MUSHROOM EGG MUFFINS

Servings: 4

Prep Time: 10 min

Cook Time: 20 min

Ingredients:

- 6 large eggs
- 1 cup of baby spinach, chop up
- 1/2 cup of mushrooms, diced
- 1/4 cup of feta cheese, crumbled
- Salt and pepper as needed
- Cooking spray

Instructions:

1. Set oven temperature to 350°F.
2. Mix eggs, diced mushrooms, chop-up spinach, crumbled feta cheese, salt, and pepper in a bowl.
3. Put cooking spray in a muffin tin and grease it.
4. Divide the egg mixture equally among the muffin cups of of of of of.
5. Bake the egg muffins for 18 to 20 min, or until they are set and have a light brown color.
6. Before removing it from the muffin tray, let cool somewhat.
7. Warm up and serve.

Nutrition Info (per serving):

Calories: 150, Protein: 12g, Carbohydrates: 2g, Fat: 10g

TURKEY AND SWEET POTATO SKILLET

Servings: 4

Prep Time: 15 min

Cook Time: 20 min

Ingredients:

- 1 lb ground turkey
- 2 sweet potatoes, peeled and diced
- 1 onion, chop-up
- 1 bell pepper, diced
- 2 cloves garlic, chop-up
- 1 tsp ground cumin
- 1 tsp smoked paprika
- Salt and pepper as needed
- 1/4 cup of fresh cilantro, chopped up

Instructions:

1. Brown the ground turkey in a large skillet over medium heat.
2. Add the chop-up garlic, diced bell pepper, diced onion, and diced sweet potatoes. Add the veggies and sauté till they soft.
3. Add salt, pepper, smoked paprika, and ground cumin for seasoning.
4. Cook the sweet potatoes for a further five to seven min, or until they are tender.
5. Before serving, garnish with fresh cilantro.
6. Warm up the food.

Nutrition Info (per serving):

Calories: 300, Protein: 25g, Carbohydrates: 25g, Fat: 10g

GREEK QUINOA SALAD

Servings: 4

Prep Time: 15 min

Cook Time: 15 min

Ingredients:

- 1 cup ofquinoa, cooked
- 1 cucumber, diced
- 1 cup of cherry tomatoes, halved
- 1/2 red onion, lightly chop-up
- 1/2 cup of Kalamata olives, split
- 1/2 cup of feta cheese, crumbled
- 1/4 cup of fresh parsley, chopped up
- 3 tbsp olive oil
- 2 tbsp red wine vinegar
- 1 tsp dried oregano
- Salt and pepper as needed

Instructions:

1. Cooked quinoa, diced cucumber, chop-up red onion, halved cherry tomatoes, split Kalamata olives, crumbled feta cheese, and chop-up fresh parsley should all be mixed in a big bowl.
2. Mix the olive oil, red wine vinegar, dried oregano, salt, and pepper in a small bowl.
3. After adding the dressing to the quinoa mixture, toss to blend.
4. Before serving, let the food cool for at least half an hour in the refrigerator.
5. Chill o serve.

Nutrition Info (per serving):

Calories: 350, Protein: 10g, Carbohydrates: 30g, Fat: 20g

BAKED EGGPLANT PARMESAN

Servings: 4

Prep Time: 20 min

Cook Time: 30 min

Ingredients:

- 2 large eggplants, split into rounds
- 2 cups of marinara sauce
- 1 cup of breadcrumbs
- 1/2 cup of finely grated Parmesan cheese
- 2 eggs, beaten
- 1 tsp dried oregano
- 1 tsp dried basil
- Salt and pepper as needed
- Fresh basil for garnish

Instructions:

1. First, butter a baking sheet and preheat the oven to 400°F.
2. Mix breadcrumbs, finely grated Parmesan cheese, dried basil, dried oregano, salt, and pepper in a shallow plate.
3. Coat the eggplant slices in the breadcrumb mixture after dipping them into beaten eggs.
4. Arrange the coated eggplant slices onto the ready baking sheet.
5. Bake the eggplant for 20 to 25 min, or until it becomes crispy and golden.
6. Arrange roasted eggplant slices, marinara sauce, and more sauce in a baking dish.
7. Bake for a further ten min.
8. Add some fresh basil as a garnish before serving.
9. Warm up the food.

Nutrition Info (per serving):

Calories: 250, Protein: 10g, Carbohydrates: 35g, Fat: 8g

CHICKEN AND BROCCOLI QUICHE

Servings: 6

Prep Time: 15 min

Cook Time: 45 min

Ingredients:

- 1 pie crust (store-bought or homemade)
- 1 cup of cooked chicken, shredded
- 1 cup of broccoli florets, steamed and chop-up
- 1 cup of shredded cheddar cheese
- 4 large eggs
- 1 cup of milk
- 1/2 tsp dried thyme
- Salt and pepper as needed

Instructions:

1. Set oven temperature to 375°F.
2. The pie crust should be rolled out and put on a pie plate.
3. Cover the pie crust with shredded cheddar cheese, chopped broccoli, and shredded chicken.
4. Mix the eggs, milk, salt, pepper, and dried thyme in a bowl.
5. Cover the chicken and broccoli in the pie crust with the egg mixture.
6. Bake the quiche for 40 to 45 min, or until it sets and the top becomes golden.
7. Before slicing, let cool slightly.
8. Warm up and serve.

Nutrition Info (per serving):

Calories: 300, Protein: 18g, Carbohydrates: 15g, Fat: 18g

PESTO SHRIMP AND ZUCCHINI NOODLES

Servings: 4

Prep Time: 15 min

Cook Time: 10 min

Ingredients:

- 1 lb large shrimp, peeled and deveined
- 3 zucchini, spiral zed into noodles
- 2 tbsp pesto sauce
- 2 tbsp olive oil
- 2 cloves garlic, chop-up
- Salt and pepper as needed
- Parmesan cheese for garnish

Instructions:

1. In a pan set over medium-high heat, heat the olive oil.
2. When aromatic, add the chop-up garlic and sauté it.
3. Cook the shrimp until they become opaque and pink.
4. Cook the zucchini noodles for two to three min, or until they are somewhat soft.
5. Mix the zucchini noodles and shrimp with the pesto sauce.
6. Add pepper and salt for seasoning.
7. Before serving, sprinkle some Parmesan cheese on top.
8. Warm up the food.

Nutrition Info (per serving):

Calories: 250, Protein: 25g, Carbohydrates: 8g, Fat: 12g

SPICY BLACK BEAN AND CORN SALSA

Servings: 6

Prep Time: 10 min

Cook Time: 0 min

Ingredients:

- 1 can of black beans that have been rinsed and drained
- 1 cup of corn kernels
- 1 cup of cherry tomatoes, halved
- 1/2 red onion, lightly chop-up
- 1 jalapeño, seeded and diced
- 1/4 cup of fresh cilantro, chopped up
- Juice of 1 lime
- Salt and pepper as needed

Instructions:

1. Black beans, corn kernels, cherry tomatoes, split jalapeño, chop-up red onion, and chop-up cilantro should all be mixed in a bowl.
2. Drizzle the mixture with one lime juice.
3. Add salt and pepper as needed, then toss to mix.
4. Let it cool for a minimum of half an hour before serving.
5. Present cold.

Nutrition Info (per serving):

Calories: 150, Protein: 6g, Carbohydrates: 28g, Fat: 1g

LEMON HERB GRILLED SWORDFISH

Servings: 4

Prep Time: 10 min

Cook Time: 10 min

Ingredients:

- 4 swordfish steaks
- Zest and juice of 1 lemon
- 2 tbsp olive oil
- 2 cloves garlic, chop-up
- 1 tsp dried oregano
- Salt and pepper as needed
- Fresh parsley for garnish

Instructions:

1. Set the grill's temperature to medium-high.
2. Mix the lemon zest, lemon juice, olive oil, dried oregano, chop-up garlic, salt, and pepper in a bowl.
3. Drizzle the swordfish steaks with the lemon-herb mixture.
4. The swordfish should be cooked through after grilling for 4–5 min on every side.
5. Before serving, garnish with fresh parsley.
6. Warm up the food.

Nutrition Info (per serving):

Calories: 300, Protein: 30g, Carbohydrates: 2g, Fat: 20g

MEDITERRANEAN STUFFED BELL PEPPERS

Servings: 4
Prep Time: 20 min
Cook Time: 30 min

Ingredients:
- 4 halved bell peppers seeds removed
- 1 cup of cooked quinoa
- 1 can (15 oz) chickpeas, drained and rinsed
- 1 cucumber, diced
- 1 cup of cherry tomatoes, halved
- 1/2 red onion, lightly chop-up
- 1/2 cup of Kalamata olives, split
- 1/2 cup of feta cheese, crumbled
- 2 tbsp olive oil
- 1 tbsp red wine vinegar
- 1 tsp dried oregano
- Salt and pepper as needed
- Fresh parsley for garnish

Instructions:
1. Set oven temperature to 375°F.
2. Cooked quinoa, chickpeas, diced cucumber, chop-up red onion, halved cherry tomatoes, split Kalamata olives, and crumbled feta cheese should all be mixed in a bowl.
3. The items needed in the dressing are red wine vinegar, dried oregano, salt, pepper, olive oil, and a small bowl.
4. After adding the dressing to the quinoa mixture, toss to blend.
5. Spoon a portion of the Mediterranean quinoa mixture into every bell pepper half.
6. Stuffed peppers should be put in a baking dish.
7. Bake the peppers for 25 to 30 min, or until they are soft.
8. Before serving, garnish with fresh parsley.
9. Warm up the food.

Nutrition Info (per serving):
Calories: 350, Protein: 10g, Carbohydrates: 35g, Fat: 18g

THAI COCONUT CURRY CHICKEN

Servings: 4

Prep Time: 15 min

Cook Time: 25 min

Ingredients:

- Cubes of one lb of skinless, boneless chicken breasts
- 1 can (14 oz) coconut milk
- 2 tbsp red curry paste
- 1 red bell pepper, split
- 1 zucchini, split
- 1 cup of snap peas
- 1 tbsp fish sauce
- 1 tbsp brown sugar
- 1 tbsp lime juice
- Fresh cilantro for garnish
- Cooked brown rice for serving

Instructions:

1. Heat the red curry paste and coconut milk in a big skillet over medium heat.
2. After adding, sauté the chicken cubes until browned.
3. Add the snap peas, zucchini, and chop-up red bell pepper, and stir.
4. Stir in lime juice, brown sugar, and fish sauce. Mix everything.
5. Simmer for 15 to 20 min, or until the chicken is cooked through and the vegetables are soft.
6. Place on top of warm brown rice.
7. Add fresh cilantro as a garnish.
8. Warm up the food.

Nutrition Info (per serving):

Calories: 350, Protein: 25g, Carbohydrates: 20g, Fat: 18g

CAPRESE CHICKEN SKEWERS

Servings: 4

Prep Time: 15 min

Cook Time: 10 min

Ingredients:

- Cubes of a lb of skinless, boneless chicken breasts
- 1 pint cherry tomatoes
- one package for pure mozzarella balls
- Fresh basil leaves
- Balsamic glaze for drizzling
- Olive oil for brushing
- Salt and pepper as needed

Instructions:

1. Turn the heat up to medium-high on the grill or grill pan.
2. Put cherry tomatoes, fresh mozzarella balls, and cubed chicken on skewers.
3. Season the skewers with salt and pepper after brushing them with olive oil.
4. Cook, rotating the chicken once or twice, for 8 to 10 min, or until cooked through.
5. Place the skewers on a plate for serving.
6. Garnish with fresh basil and drizzle with balsamic glaze.
7. Warm up the food.

Nutrition Info (per serving):

Calories: 300, Protein: 30g, Carbohydrates: 5g, Fat: 18g

CAULIFLOWER AND CHICKPEA CURRY

Servings: 4

Prep Time: 15 min

Cook Time: 25 min

Ingredients:

- 1 cauliflower, cut into florets
- 1 can (15 oz) chickpeas, drained and rinsed
- 1 onion, chop-up
- 2 cloves garlic, chop-up
- 1 can (14 oz) coconut milk
- 1 can (14 oz) diced tomatoes
- 2 tbsp curry powder
- 1 tsp ground turmeric
- 1 tsp ground cumin
- Salt and pepper as needed
- Fresh cilantro for garnish
- Cooked basmati rice for serving

Instructions:

1. Diced onion and chopped garlic should be cooked in a big pot until they are tender.
2. Add the chickpeas and cauliflower florets to the pot.
3. Add the diced tomatoes, coconut milk, curry powder, cumin, turmeric, and salt & pepper as needed.
4. Simmer until the cauliflower is soft, 20 to 25 min.
5. Accompany with cooked basmati rice.
6. Add fresh cilantro as a garnish.
7. Warm up the food.

Nutrition Info (per serving):

Calories: 350, Protein: 15g, Carbohydrates: 30g, Fat: 20g

TURKEY AND SPINACH STUFFED MUSHROOMS

Servings: 4

Prep Time: 20 min

Cook Time: 20 min

Ingredients:

- 16 large mushrooms, stems removed and chop up
- 1 lb ground turkey
- 1 onion, lightly chop-up
- 2 cloves garlic, chop-up
- 1 cup of baby spinach, chop up
- 1/2 cup of breadcrumbs
- • 1/4 cup of Parmesan cheese which is roughly grated
- 1 tsp dried thyme
- Salt and pepper as needed
- Olive oil for brushing

Instructions:

1. Set oven temperature to 375°F.
2. Chop-up mushroom stems, ground turkey, chop-up onion, and chop-up garlic should all be sautéed in a skillet until the meat is browned.
3. Cook the baby spinach till it wilts by adding it chopped up.
4. Add breadcrumbs, salt, pepper, dried thyme, and finely grated Parmesan cheese.
5. After brushing the mushroom caps with olive oil, stuff them with the mixture of spinach and turkey.
6. Stuffed mushrooms ought to be put on a baking pan.
7. Bake mushrooms for 15 to 20 min, or until they are soft.
8. Warm up the food.

Nutrition Info (per serving):

Calories: 250, Protein: 20g, Carbohydrates: 15g, Fat: 12g

ASIAN SESAME SALMON BOWL

Servings: 4

Prep Time: 15 min

Cook Time: 15 min

Ingredients:

- 4 salmon fillets
- 1 cup of broccoli florets
- 1 carrot, julienned
- 1 bell pepper, split
- 2 cups of cooked brown rice
- 2 tbsp soy sauce
- 1 tbsp sesame oil
- 1 tbsp rice vinegar
- 1 tbsp honey
- 1 tsp ginger, finely grated
- 1 tsp sesame seeds
- Green onions for garnish

Instructions:

1. Set oven temperature to 400°F.
2. Salmon fillets should be put on a baking pan.
3. Arrange the split bell pepper, julienned carrot, and broccoli florets around the fish.
4. Mix soy sauce, sesame oil, rice vinegar, honey, and finely grated ginger in a bowl.
5. Apply the soy sauce mixture to the fish and vegetables.
6. Bake the salmon for 12 to 15 min, or until it is cooked through.
7. Place on top of warm brown rice.
8. Add a drizzle of any leftover sauce, green onions, and sesame seeds as garnish.
9. Warm up the food.

Nutrition Info (per serving):

Calories: 400, Protein: 30g, Carbohydrates: 40g, Fat: 15g

ZUCCHINI AND CORN FRITTERS

Servings: 4

Prep Time: 15 min

Cook Time: 15 min

Ingredients:

- 2 cup of zucchini, finely grated
- 1 cup of corn kernels (fresh or frozen)
- 1/2 cup of whole wheat flour
- 1/4 cup of Parmesan cheese which was heavily grated
- 2 green onions, lightly chop-up
- 2 eggs, beaten
- 1 tsp baking powder
- Salt and pepper as needed
- Olive oil for frying

Instructions:

1. Finely grated zucchini, corn kernels, whole wheat flour, finely grated Parmesan cheese, chop-up green onions, beaten eggs, baking powder, salt, and pepper should all be mixed in a big basin.
2. In a skillet over medium heat, warm the olive oil.
3. Spoonfuls of batter should be dropped into the skillet and smoothed with the back of a spoon.
4. Cook till golden brown, 3–4 min on every side.
5. blot with paper towels.
6. Warm up the food.

Nutrition Info (per serving):

Calories: 200, Protein: 8g, Carbohydrates: 25g, Fat: 8g

CONCLUSION

More significantly, congrats on making an investment in your health, your quest toward long-term fitness, and yourself by finishing the last pages of the Weight Loss Recipe Book for Watchers 2025.

You have learned how eating can be both pleasant and nourishing throughout this cookbook, how making modest changes may have a big impact, and how the secret to long-term weight loss is to be consistent rather than perfect. You've learned that eating healthily just means learning to make more intelligent, thoughtful decisions rather than sacrificing taste, happiness, or your favorite foods.

Every action you've performed moves you closer to your objectives, whether it was trying a single new recipe or adding new ideas to your weekly rotation. You now know how to easily prepare balanced meals, stay on track even when life gets hectic, and take advantage of SmartPointsTM and ZeroPointsTM foods. Above all, you have demonstrated to yourself that you are capable of doing this, one meal, one day, and one choice at a time.

Keep in mind that progress is a personal journey as you proceed. It's not necessary for your journey to resemble anyone else's. Honor each victory, no matter how tiny.

You're forming lifelong habits. Every recipe you make is a step toward long-term wellbeing and self-care.

No one is "perfect." All that has to be done is to show up, learn, adapt, and carry on in a friendly and reliable manner.

Make this book a go-to source for you anytime you need motivation, support, or a tasty WW-friendly dinner. Allow your kitchen to be a room where you support your objectives, take care of your health, and savor every bite—a place of empowerment rather than pressure.

We appreciate you include this cookbook in your trip. Cheers to a year of living lighter, stronger, and happier than ever before, to food that satisfies and fuels, and to your continuing success.

Printed in Dunstable, United Kingdom